The Originality of Super Foods

Disclaimer

This e-book has been written for information purposes only. Every effort has been made to make this ebook as complete and accurate as possible.

However, there may be mistakes in typography or content. Also, this ebook provides information only up to the publishing date. Therefore, this ebook should be used as a guide - not as the ultimate source.
The purpose of this ebook is to educate. The author and the publisher does not warrant that the information contained in this e-book is fully complete and shall not be responsible for any errors or omissions.

The author and publisher shall have neither liability nor responsibility to any person or entity with respect to any loss or damage caused or alleged to be caused directly or indirectly by this ebook.

Table of Content

Introductory

We all hear about the many wonderful foods that are good to eat, and good for us. We always hear about eating fruits, and vegetables, and nuts.

But that's a big list to sort through, and wouldn't it be simpler to have a few super foods that you can always turn to? To help you in your endeavors to lead a healthy lifestyle and a healthy life you can use the list compiled below as quick reference list of 9 super foods. These super foods and 14 others can be found in Superfoods Health-Style, by Steven G. Pratt M.D.

Apples

Apples are a great food for many reasons including the ability to reduce the risk or heart disease, certain cancers, high blood pressure, and type-2 diabetes. They also benefit the respiratory system by preventing lung cancer and asthma.

By consuming apples your body gets fiber, potassium and antioxidants, such as Vitamin C and polyphenols. Studies show that the real benefit comes from the synergistic interaction between these ingredients.

To take best advantage of apples for your health, eat a wide variety and make sure that you eat the peel, which contains several times more antioxidants than the inside. As they say, eat an apple a day.

Avocados

When you want to help your body absorb more nutrients from the foods you eat, have an avocado too. Fat soluble phytonutrients, like beta-carotene, are more easily absorbed by the body because of the monounsaturated fat in the avocado.

Avocados also help you keep your weight down because they help you feel full, which triggers your body to stop eating. They are calorie rich at 48 calories per ounce, so for best results eat one-third to one-half an avocado two to three times a week.

Dark Chocolate

When you want a little indulgence with your health food, try dark chocolate. It contains lots of polyphenols which lower blood pressure and is a natural anti-inflammatory. You should keep in mind that blood pressure lowering qualities are only in dark chocolate, but not in its cousin, milk chocolate.

In 2000 a study published by the American Journal of Clinical Nutrition showed that the effect on blood flow from high flavanol cocoa was similar to taking a low-dose aspirin. These means that dark chocolate could possibly be used to treat ailments like minor pains or headaches.

For the best results use Newman's Own Sweet Dart Chocolate, as Dr Pratt has found it has more polyphenols than any other dark chocolate he has found. Like avocado, chocolate is high in calories, so shoot for no more than 100 calories a day.

Olive Oil

There has been much discussion lately about the benefits of the Mediterranean diet. Well olive oil is one of the main components of that diet and its benefits are outstanding. It is a great substitute for other oils and fats and has been shown to reduce the risk of breast and colon cancer, lower blood pressure, and improve the health of your cardiovascular system.

For best results take a tablespoon a day of extra virgin olive oil that is cold pressed and greenish in color. This green color helps you spot high levels of polyphenols.

Garlic

Another component of the Mediterranean diet, Garlic is great for your cardiovascular system. By eating garlic regularly, you can reduce your blood pressure, triglyceride levels and your LDL(bad) cholesterol. Garlic also has anti-inflammatory agents and antibiotic properties.

To grab all the health benefits of garlic, eat one clove several times a week. Raw garlic is best, but cooked is good too. Keep in mind that dried garlic and garlic supplements don't have the same benefits as fresh garlic.

Honey

Honey is not often seen on many lists of healthy foods, but don't let that fool you. Eating honey daily increases the amounts of antioxidant in the blood, helps to prevent constipation, and reduces cholesterol and blood pressure.

If you are running low on energy, reach for the honey, not sugar. Honey does a better job of maintaining blood sugar and energy than other sweeteners. And choose dark honeys over light ones, because they are higher in antioxidants and flavor. One to two teaspoons several times a week should do the trick.

Kiwis

If you want extreme quantities of Vitamin C and E that can reduce risk of asthma, osteoarthritis, and colon cancer, and boost your immune system, then grab a kiwi or two. An interesting point to keep in mind is that dietary vitamin E appears to lower the risk of Alzheimer's, and by consuming kiwis, you get vitamin E without the calories that most other vitamin e rich foods contain, like nuts and oils.

Another stellar ingredient is lutein, which lowers the risk cataracts and macular degeneration. To get all the above benefits and reduce the risk of blood clots, then consume one kiwi, two to three times a week.

Onions

For the benefits of onions, you can just reread the benefits of garlic, because they are pretty much the same.

Try to eat dishes containing onions at least three times a week, and make sure that you let the onion sit for 5 to 10 minutes after you cut it open. If you apply heat too soon you will deactivate the thiopropanal sulfoxide, which is the substance in the onion that gives us the most heart benefits. And remember the more pungent the onion, the better it is for you.
Pomegranates

Pomegranates are packed with tons of phytochemicals like potassium, which is great for lowering your blood pressure. Studies also suggest that pomegranates can slow the progression of prostate cancer and reduce the risk of atherosclerosis.

Instead of fighting with the little pulpy seeds to get your dose of pomegranate, try four to eight ounces of 100% juice several times a week. Be sure to stay away from juices with added sugar.

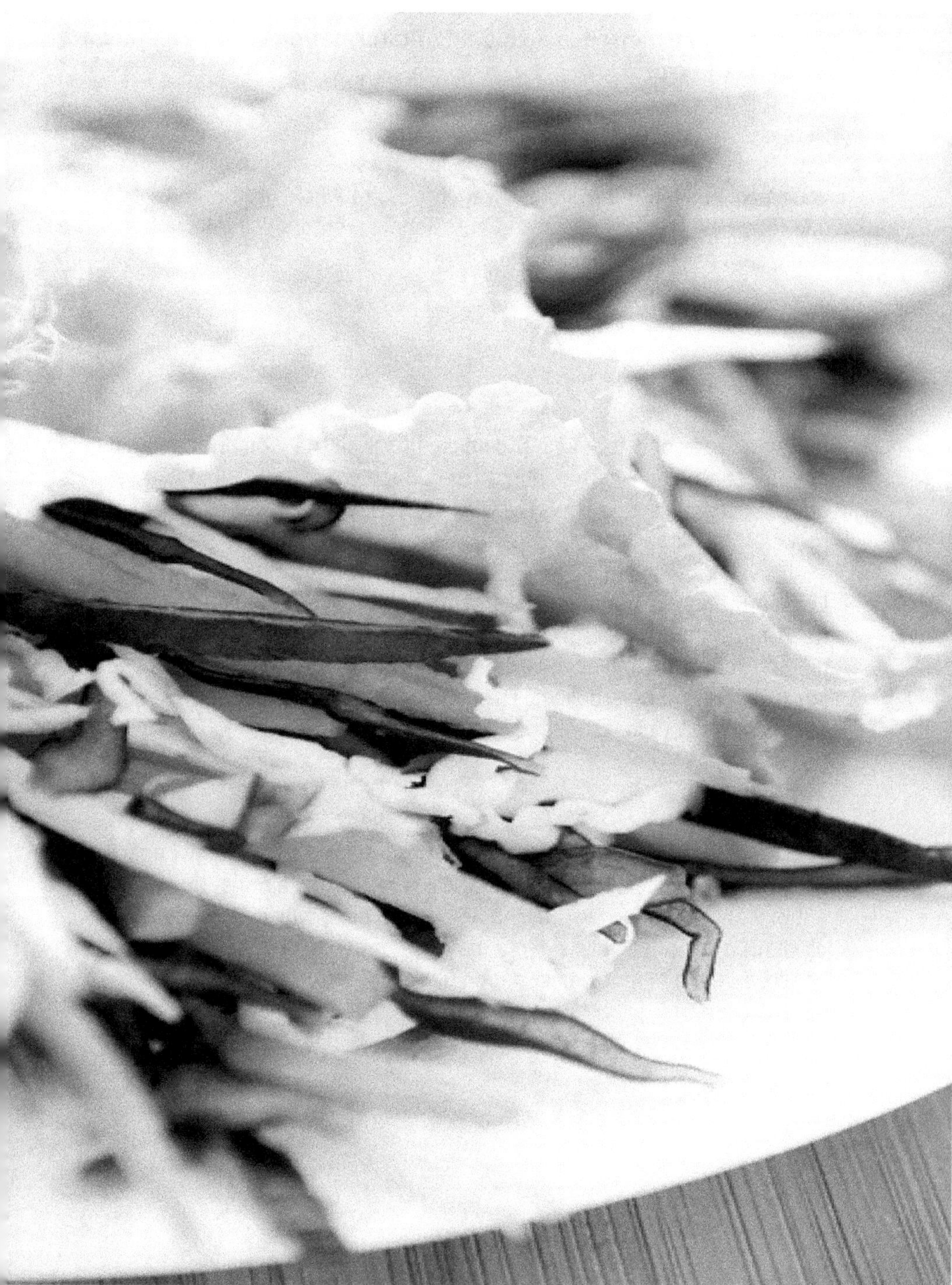

Chapter 1: Nutrition - The Super Foods That Keep You Healthy

Get ready to experience a volume of information of the healthiest foods in the world.

Here is a list of the top ten super foods that most health experts agree on. You should tell everyone you know about these foods and enjoy them at your next meal. From fruits and vegetables, to whole grains, nuts, beans and legumes, this power-packed nutritional inventory will take you into the best years of your life and beyond.

Fruits

1. Cantaloupe

Only a quarter of cantaloupe provides almost all the vitamin A needed in one day. Since the beta-carotene in a cantaloupe converts to vitamin A, you get both nutrients at once. These vision-strengthening nutrients may help reduce the risk of developing cataracts.

Like an orange, cantaloupe is also an excellent source of vitamin C, which helps our immune system. It is also being a good source of vitamin B6, dietary fiber, folate, niacin, and potassium, which helps maintain good blood sugar levels and metabolism. This pale orange power fruit may help reduce our risk of heart disease, stroke, and cancer.

2. Blueberries

These mildly sweet (and sometimes tangy) berries offer a high capacity to destroy free radicals that can cause cancer. Low in calories, they offer antioxidant phytonutrients called anthocyanidins, which enhance the effects of vitamin C. These antioxidants may help prevent cataracts, glaucoma, varicose veins, hemorrhoids, peptic ulcers, heart disease and cancer.

Vegetables

3: Tomatoes

Tomatoes help us fight against heart disease and cancers such as colorectal, prostate, breast, endometrial, lung, and cancer of the pancreas. Tomatoes are also good sources of vitamin C, A, and K. In a 2004 study, it was found that tomato juice alone can help reduce blood clotting.

Fresh, organic tomatoes deliver three times as much of the cancer-fighting carotenoid lycopene. Even organic ketchup is better for you than regular ketchup! Look for tomato paste's and sauces that contain the whole tomato (including peels) because you will absorb 75% more lycopene and almost two times the amount of beta-carotene.

4: Sweet Potatoes

As an excellent source of vitamin, A, C, and manganese, sweet potatoes are also a good source of copper, dietary fiber, vitamin B6, potassium and iron. Those who are smokers or prone to second- hand smoke may benefit greatly from this root vegetable that helps protect us against emphysema.

For a unique dessert, cube a cooked sweet potato and slice a banana. Then lightly pour maple syrup over the top and add a dash or two of cinnamon. Add chopped walnuts for an even healthier kick.

5: Spinach and Kale

A cancer-fighter and cardio-helper, spinach and kale top the list as far as green leafy vegetables are concerned. Much like broccoli, they provide an excellent source of vitamin A and C. Kale is a surprisingly good source of calcium at 25% per cup, boiled. Vitamin K is abundantly found in spinach as well, with almost 200% of the Daily Value available, to help reduce bone loss.

Whole Grains

6: Whole Grain Bread, Pasta and Brown Rice

Whether it's bread or pasta, the first thing to check for when purchasing whole grain bread and pasta is to make sure it is 100% whole grain.

Remember to check the list of ingredients on the package. For example, look for the exact phrase "whole wheat flour" as one of the first ingredients listed in whole wheat bread. If it's not listed as such, then it's not whole grain. Wheat bran is a cancer-fighting grain that also helps us regulate our bowel movements.

Brown rice is also a better choice than refined grain (white rice) for the same reason as choosing whole wheat bread. Whole wheat flour or brown rice that turns into white flour or white rice actually destroys between 50-90% of vitamin B3, vitamin B1, vitamin B6, manganese, phosphorus, iron, and all of the dietary fiber and essential fatty acids we need.

Even when processed white flour or white rice is "enriched," it is not in the same form as the original unprocessed kind. In fact, 11 nutrients are actually lost and are not replaced during the "enrichment" process!

Nuts

7: Walnuts

These nuts are packed with omega-3 fats, which is one of the "good" fats. A quarter cup of walnuts would take care of about 90% of the omega-3s needed in one day. Walnuts provide many health benefits including cardiovascular protection, better cognitive function, anti-inflammatory advantages relating to asthma, rheumatoid arthritis, and inflammatory skin diseases like eczema and psoriasis. They can even help against cancer and also support the immune system.

Beans and Legumes

8: Black Beans and Lentils

While black beans are a good source of fiber that can lower cholesterol, so are lentils. The high fiber content in both black beans and lentils helps to maintain blood sugar levels. Also, a fat-free, high quality protein with additional minerals and B-vitamins, black beans and lentils fill you up and don't expand your waistline.

A complete, one-stop source of using a variety of beans and lentils comes easy when you can find a bag of 15-bean mix (includes black beans, lentils, navy, pinto, red, kidney, etc.) at the grocery store. Consider making a delicious soup with the addition of tomatoes, onions, garlic and your favorite spices with this bean mixture.

Dairy

9: Skim Milk and Yogurt

Skim milk (or low-fat) helps to promote strong bones, offering an excellent source of calcium, vitamin D, and vitamin K. These nutrients help protect colon cells from cancer-causing chemicals, bone loss, migraine headaches, premenstrual symptoms, and childhood obesity. Recent studies also show that overweight adults lose weight, especially around the midsection, when consuming low-fat dairy such as skim milk and yogurt.

Yogurt also includes the essential nutrients such as phosphorous and vitamin B2, vitamin B12, vitamin B5, zinc, potassium, and protein. Yogurt's live bacterial cultures also provide a wealth of health benefits that may help us live longer and strengthen our immune system.

Seafood

10: Salmon

Salmon is high in protein, low in saturated fat and high in omega-3 fats (the essential fatty acids that are also found in those walnuts mentioned earlier). Salmon is a heart-healthy food and is recommended to eat at least twice a week.

When choosing salmon, it's best to stay away from farm raised and select wild instead. Research studies show that farmed salmon may cause cancer because it may carry high levels of carcinogenic chemicals known as polychlorinated biphenyls (PCBs).

Others

Green Tea and "Power" Water

Although not food per say, the health benefits of these beverages are worthy of mentioning.

Green tea has beneficial phytonutrients and lower levels of caffeine than all other teas. The more research studying green tea, the more health benefits are found. A cancer fighter as well, green tea has antioxidant effects that lower risks of bacterial or viral infections to cardiovascular disease, cancer, stroke, periodontal disease, and osteoporosis.

Water packed with vitamins and/or naturally sweetened fruit are also the newest trend. Some offer a full day's supply of vitamin C while others promise no artificial sweeteners with a full, fruity taste.

As you can see, the top ten super foods are worth every bite (or sip). Now that you know which foods can help save your life, what's more important than investing in your health?

Chapter 2: You Really Are What You Eat

Recent dietary research has uncovered 14 different nutrient-dense foods that time and again promote good overall health.

Coined "superfoods," they tend to have fewer calories, higher levels of vitamins and minerals, and many disease-fighting antioxidants.

Beans (legumes), berries (especially blueberries), broccoli, green tea, nuts (especially walnuts), oranges, pumpkin, salmon, soy, spinach, tomatoes, turkey, whole grains and oats, and yogurt can all help stop and even reverse diseases such as hypertension, diabetes, Alzheimer's, and some forms of cancer.

And where one might have an effect on a certain part of the body, it can also affect the health of other body functions and performance, since the whole body is connected.

With these 14 foods as the base of a balanced, solid diet, weight loss gimmicks and other fly-by-night programs can become a thing of the past in your life.

Conversely, the ill-effects of an unbalanced diet are several and varied. Low energy levels, mood swings, tired all the time, weight change, uncomfortable with body are just a few signs that your diet is unbalanced. An unbalanced diet can cause problems with maintenance of body tissues, growth and development, brain and nervous system function, as well as problems with bone and muscle systems.

Symptoms of malnutrition include lack of energy, irritability, a weakened immune system leading to frequent colds or allergies, and mineral depletion that can trigger a variety of health concerns including anemia.

And since the body is connected, realizing that an unhealthy body will result in an unhealthy spirit only makes sense. When we nourish our body with these superfoods and complement them with other nutrient-dense and healthy fresh foods, our spirit will be vitalized and healthy as a direct result.

Many modern diets based on prepackaged convenience foods are sorely lacking in many vitamins and minerals, which can affect our mental capacities as well, and cause irritability, confusion, and the feeling of 'being in a fog' all the time.

Superfoods can be the basis of a sound, healthy, nutritious solution to curing many of these ailments and more.

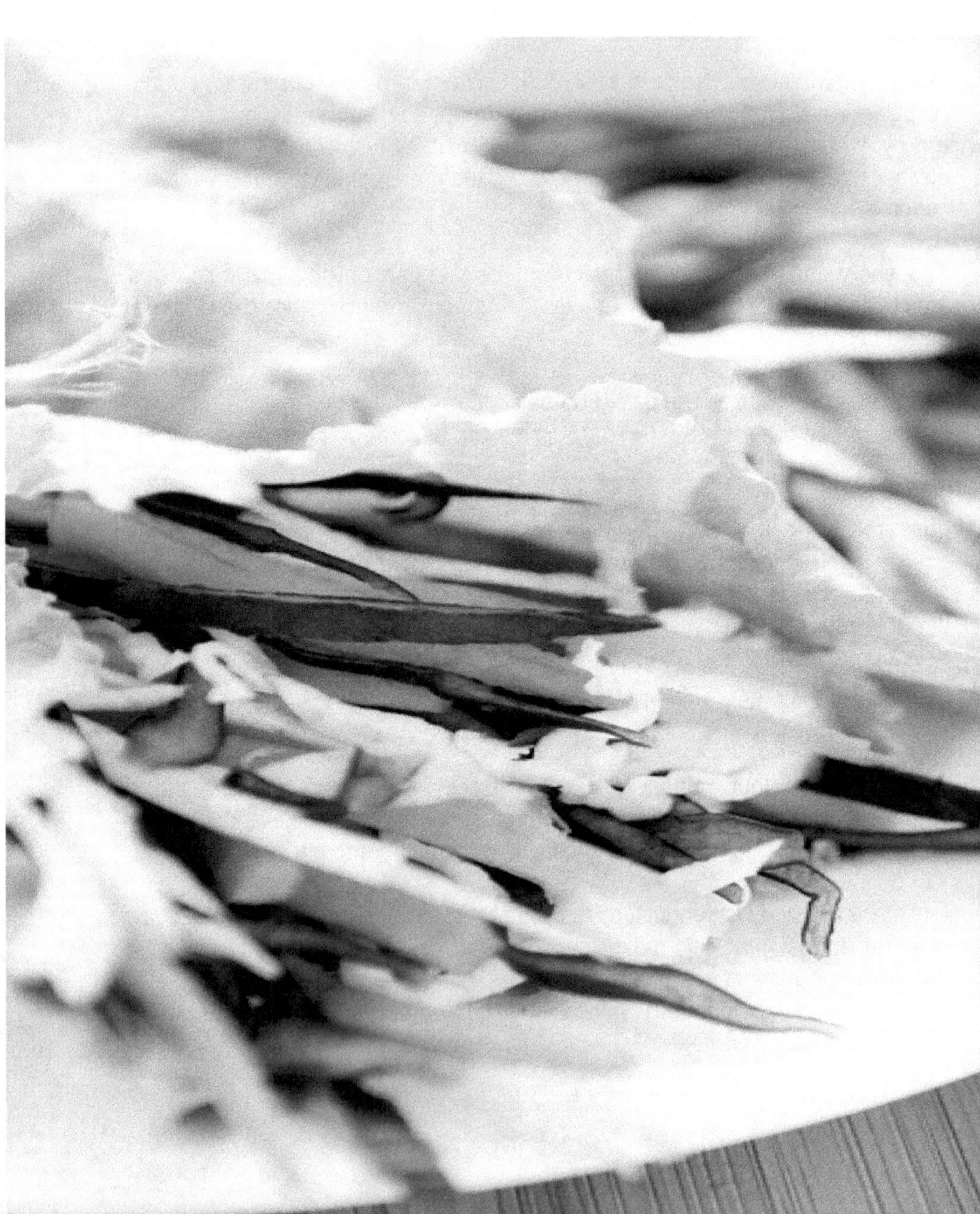

Chapter 3: Color Your Way to Daily Health

It's important that we eat plenty of different fruits and vegetables every day.

Diets rich in fruits and vegetables may reduce the risk of cancer and other chronic diseases. Fruits and vegetables provide essential vitamins and minerals, fiber, and other substances that are important for good health. Most fruits and vegetables are naturally low in fat and calories and are filling.

You've probably heard about the 5 A Day for Better Health program. It provides easy ways to add more fruits and vegetables into your daily eating patterns. It's vital that we eat a wide variety of colorful orange/yellow, red, green, white, and blue/purple vegetables and fruit every day.

By eating vegetables and fruit from each color group, you will benefit from the essential vitamins, minerals, and fiber that each color group has to offer alone and in combination.

There's several different yet simple ways to start incorporating vegetables and fruit into your familiar and favorite meals. You can begin your day with 100 percent fruit or vegetable juice, slice bananas or strawberries on top of your cereal, or have a salad with lunch and an apple for an afternoon snack.

Include a vegetable with dinner and you already have about 5 cups of fruits and vegetables. You may even try adding a piece of fruit for a snack or an extra vegetable at dinner.

Don't be afraid to try something new to increase your vegetable and fruit intake. There are so many choices when selecting fruits and vegetables. Kiwifruit, asparagus, and mango may become your new favorite. Keep things fresh and interesting by combining fruits and vegetables of different flavors and colors, like red grapes with pineapple chunks, or cucumbers and red peppers.

Get in the habit of keeping fruits and vegetables visible and easily accessible – you'll tend to eat them more. Store cut and cleaned produce at eye-level in the refrigerator, or keep a big colorful bowl of fruit on the table.

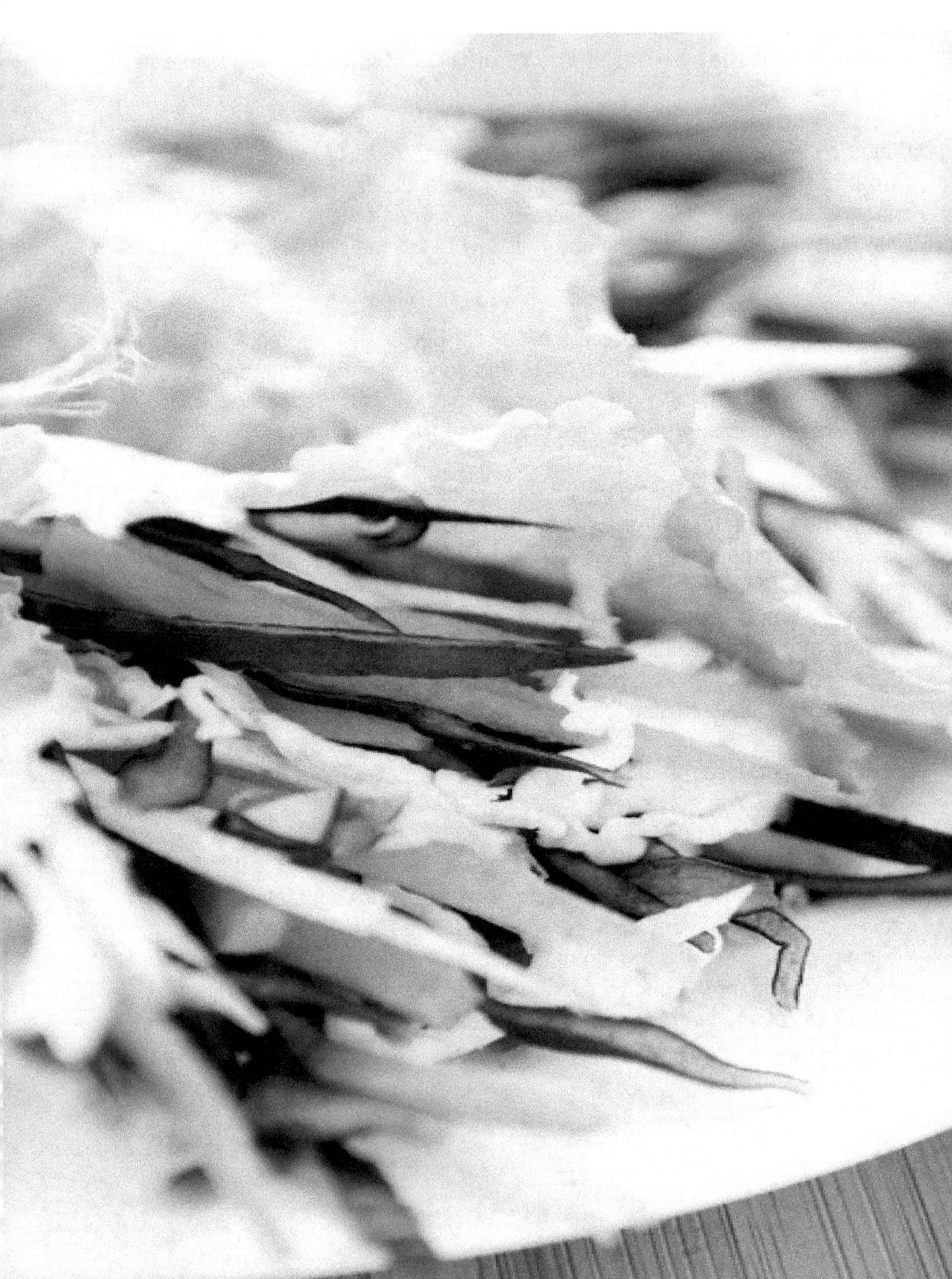

Chapter 4: Superfoods For Age-Defying Beauty

This article explores the World's Top 6 superfoods for ultimate age-defying beauty.

6 superfoods for age-defying beauty:

1) Goji Berries

Goji berries, Hollywood's hottest new food, are one of the most nutritionally dense foods on earth and house a staggering concentration of vitamins, minerals, amino acids, phytochemicals and essential fatty acids. With such an awesome constitution it is not surprising they are reputed anti-aging marvels.

Originating in Tibet and greatly favored in traditional medicine these dried berries have many noted health benefits including boosting immunity, lowering cholesterol, enhancing vision, fighting cancer cells, relieving depression and aiding weight loss.

Goji berries contain 500 times more vitamin C than oranges by weight and more beta-carotene than carrots making them a superb source of vitamin A. Together with vitamin E and essential fatty acids, these berries are ideal for any anti-aging and beauty regime.

They also contain polysaccharides, one of which has been found to stimulate the secretion of the rejuvenating human growth hormone by the pituitary gland, as well as B vitamins, 21 minerals and 18 amino acids.

The most well documented case of longevity is that of Li Qing Yuen, who lived to the age of 252. Born in 1678, he is said to have married 14 times with 11 generations of posterity before his death in 1930. Li Qing Yuen reportedly consumed goji berries daily.

A study cited in Dr. Mindell's book 'Goji: The Himalayan Health Secret', observed that 67 per cent of elderly people that were given a daily dose of the berries for 3 weeks experienced dramatic immune system enhancement and a significant improvement in spirit and optimism.

2) Aloe Vera

Forget Botox, Aloe Vera increases collagen production 100% naturally for a youthful, wrinkle-free complexion and plump, beautiful skin. The ultimate Botox alternative!

The inner gel of the Aloe versa leaf contains around 200 active compounds with over 75 nutrients. These include 20 minerals, 18 amino acids and 12 vitamins (even vitamin B12 – one of the very few plant sources of this vitamin).

Aloe Vera also has anti-microbial properties fighting fungi and bacteria and houses anti-inflammatory plant steroids and enzymes. Aloe Vera is known to aid digestion and elimination, boost the immune system, and be highly effective at healing, moisturizing and rejuvenating the skin, naturally stimulating the production of collagen.

Aloe Vera is best eaten fresh when possible (you can order large Aloe Vera leaves which last a few weeks refrigerated). Scrape out the inside gel, avoiding the outside of the leaf which is a strong laxative, and blend with fruit for the ultimate beautifying smoothie. Aloe Vera has a mild flavor though a slight bitter edge, hence is best combined with fruit.

3) Avocados

Avocados are smoothing and softening for the skin and easily absorbed; compared with almond, corn, olive, and soybean oils, avocado oil has the highest skin penetration rate.

Avocado also contains vitamin E (excellent for the skin), antioxidant carotenoids and the master antioxidant glutathione that is exceptionally powerful and has anti-carcinogenic potential. High levels of glutathione are found in the liver where the elimination of toxic materials takes place.

Glutathione is effective against pollutants such as cigarette smoke and exhaust fumes as well as ultra-violet radiation. Research is currently exploring the potential benefits of glutathione for numerous conditions including cancer, heart disease, memory loss, arthritis, Parkinson's disease, eczema, liver disorders, heavy metal poisoning and AIDS.

4) Chlorella

The nucleic acids RNA and DNA in Chlorella (one of the highest known sources of such) direct cellular growth and repair and enable our bodies to utilize nutrients more effectively, eliminate toxins and avoid disease.

The production of nucleic acids in the body declines progressively as we age, which is no doubt why their intake is recommended by Dr. Benjamin Frank in 'The No-Aging Diet'.

Paul Pitchford in 'Healing with Whole Foods' writes that 'insufficient nucleic acid causes premature aging as well as weakened immunity', Research at the Medical College of Kanazawa in Japan found that mice that were fed chlorella had a 30 per cent increase in life span. Replenishing RNA and DNA can be key to overall health, immunity and longevity.

In addition to nucleic acids, chlorella is jam-packed with vitamins, minerals, antioxidants, enzymes and amino acids, making it an incredibly rejuvenating and health-promoting superfood. Spirulina is a virtuous equivalent.

5) Bee pollen

When it comes to young and beautiful skin, bee pollen has outstanding gifts. Swedish dermatologist Dr. Lars-Erik Essen uses bee pollen to successfully treat acne and other skin conditions and observes it's beautifying and anti-aging effects.

He reports that bee pollen 'seems to prevent premature aging of the cells and stimulates growth of new skin tissue. It offers effective protection against dehydration and injects new life into dry cells. It smoothest away wrinkles and stimulates a life-giving blood supply to all skin cells.'

He believes it's skin rejuvenation properties are due to its high concentration of nucleic acids RNA and DNA, as well as its natural antibiotic action. Bee pollen has a host of other health-promoting benefits that include fighting infections, lowering cholesterol, strengthening the blood, Boosting the immune system, increasing physical strength and stamina, aiding longevity and enhancing libido! It has been called a 'prefect food' because it is so nutritionally complete.

6) Coconut oil

Coconut oil speeds up your metabolism and can actually help you loose weight. It is also incredibly beautifying and moisturizing for the skin and has antioxidant properties which protect against free-radical damage, keeping the skin youthful and healthy

Taken internally or externally coconut oil is a great ally for any beauty skin care regime. It also contains lauric acid, an anti-microbial fatty acid that kills bacteria, viruses and fungi.

Chapter 5: Superfoods for a Super Long Life

Recent research shows that specific chemicals in foods -- such as sulforaphane, a phytochemical in broccoli -- work with your genes to ratchet up your body's natural defense systems, helping to inactivate toxins and free radicals before they can do the damage that leads to cancer, cardiovascular disease, and even premature aging.

And the hope for the future is to be able to tell someone what diseases or maladies they are might be genetically predisposition to early on, so their diets can be focused accordingly.

We'll know which ones to add, which ones to avoid, and be able to take a proactive role in preventing or deterring a genetic disease. In the meantime, many foods have been determined to pack a punch to the aging process.

Lycopene, the pigment that makes tomatoes red, also appears to reduce risk for cardiovascular disease, some cancers, and macular degeneration. It's also been associated in greater self-sufficiency in elderly adults.

While fresh tomatoes have a good hit of lycopene, the most absorbable forms are found in cooked tomato products, such as spaghetti sauce and soup and prepared salsas. Pink grapefruit, guava, red bell peppers, and watermelon are also rich in lycopene.

Eating at least two cups of orange fruits like sweet potatoes, squash and carrots boosts intake of beta-carotene, which converts to vitamin A, essential for healthy skin and eyes, and which may also reduce the risk of some cancers, cardiovascular disease, and osteoporosis.

Lutein and lycopene, also found in orange produce, also help reduce the risk of macular degeneration and may protect skin from sun damage and even reduce wrinkling as well. Mangos and cantaloupes are also beta-carotene endowed.

And if you don't do anything else to change your diet, eat your dark leafy greens. They have been showed to significantly reduce your risk for heart disease and may also save your eyesight. Dietary guidelines advise at least three cups of greens a week. Frozen or bagged is as good as fresh.

Don't forget the mental aging process either. The heart-healthy omega 3 fatty acids have also recently been shown to keep your brain sharp. A recent study found that a higher intake of fatty fish significantly reduced mental decline. If fresh fish isn't an option, go for canned tuna, salmon, and sardines.

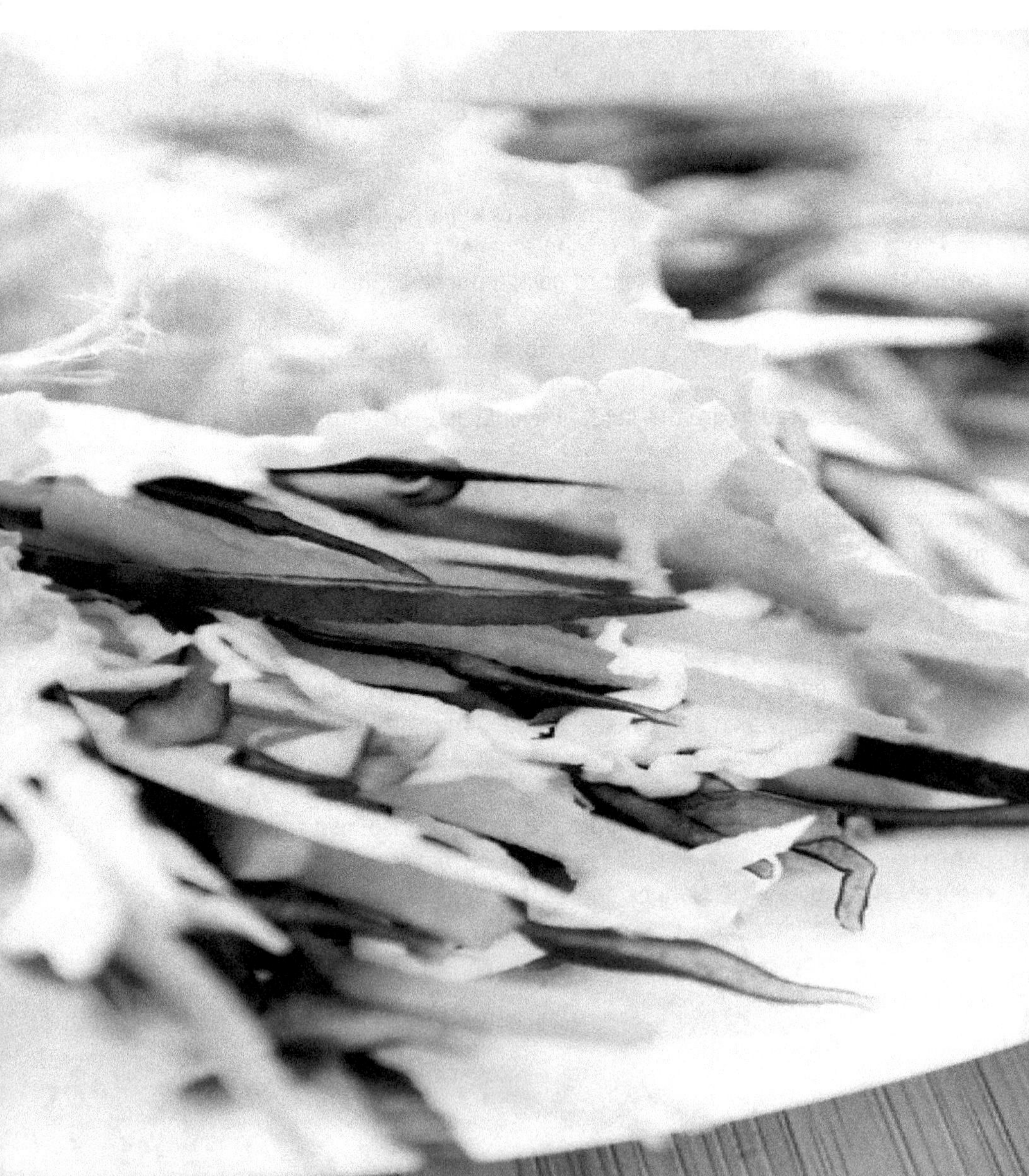

Chapter 6: Superfoods for Super Skin

It's been said we are what we eat, and that sentiment definitely holds true when it comes to our skin.

It's our body's biggest organ, and it deserves all the nutritional TLC we can give it. So, take a look at what you've been feeding yourself, and therefore feeding your skin.

One the most important components of skin health is vitamin A, and probably one of the best sources of it is low-fat dairy products. It could be said the health of our skin depends on vitamin A.

Low-fat yogurt is not only high in vitamin A, but also acidophilus, the "live" bacteria that is good for intestinal health. Turns out, it may also have an impact on the skin, since it aids in digestion. Other good sources of vitamin A include cod liver oil, sweet potatoes, carrots, leafy vegetables, and fortified breakfast cereals.

It's important to also make sure you're eating foods rich in antioxidants, such as blackberries, blueberries, strawberries, and plums. The benefits of these foods for healthy skin are plentiful. The antioxidants and other phytochemicals in these fruits can protect the skin cells, so there is less chance for damage.

This in turn guards against premature aging, and keeps skin looking younger longer. Other fruits and vegetables that are high in antioxidants include artichokes, black, red, and pinto beans, prunes, and pecans.

Essential fatty acids (EFAs) are essential to your skin. Include salmon, walnuts, canola oil, and flax seed. EFAs keep cell membranes healthy, and allow nutrients to pass through.

We also need healthy oils, which contain more than essential fatty acids. Eating good-quality oils helps keep skin lubricated and keeps it looking and feeling healthier overall. Look for oils that are cold pressed, such as olive or extra virgin oil. We only need about two tablespoons a day of healthy oils, so use wisely.

Selenium plays an important role in the health of skin cells. Turn to foods like Whole-wheat bread, muffins, and cereals; turkey, tuna and brazil nuts for this important nutrient. Recent studies show that if selenium levels are high, even skin damaged by the sun may only suffer minimal, if any, damage.

Choosing the whole grain versions of complex carbohydrates can have a significant effect on insulin levels. Processed and refined sugars can cause inflammation that may ultimately be linked to skin break outs.

Green tea has anti-inflammatory properties, and it protects the membrane of the cell. It may even help prevent or reduce skin cancer risks.

Water plays such an important role in your overall health, and it has a profound effect on your skin's health as well. Well-hydrated skin is healthy and young-looking. It also helps move the toxins out of your system so they have less chance to do damage.

Chapter 7: Superfoods that Squash Stress

Life has a way of getting the best of us some days. Whether it's working too many hours, shuffling your kids all over town for their activities, taking care of your household, or dealing with personal or family matters, stress can take its toll on you physically, mentally, emotionally, and spiritually.

But there are simple steps you can take to combat stress, starting with the foods you eat.

Avoiding caffeine and alcohol is a good start when life's particularly stressful. Stimulants and depressants like these can both zap your energy and rob you of the fuel you need to successfully cope with tension. Sugary foods should also be avoided as well, as they cause your blood sugar levels to spike then dip rapidly, which can in turn make your energy levels spike and dip at the same rate.

However, there are several superfoods out there that provide you with the energy and nutrition your body needs to keep stress in check

Asparagus, which is high in folic acid, can help level out your moods. Folic acid and vitamin B are key players in producing serotonin, a chemical that gets you into a good mood.

And though we may hear negative things regarding red meat, it's actually a wise dinner option for a stressed-out family. Beef's high levels of iron, zinc and B vitamins not only help get you into a good mood, but help you stay there as well. Your local butcher can help you select lean cuts for the healthiest options

Milk really does a body good. Chock full of calcium, protein, antioxidants, and vitamins B2 and B12, it helps strengthen bones and promotes healthy cell regeneration.

Paired with a healthy whole-grain cereal choice in the morning, low-fat milk is a great way to start your day and arm yourself to do battle with the stressors that await you. Cottage cheese is also another great dairy choice, and when coupled with a fruit that's high in vitamin C, it helps the body battle free radicals that run rampant during your most stressed periods.

Almonds are also an awesome choice when it comes to arming yourself against stress. They're high in magnesium, zinc, as well as vitamins B2, C, and E and unsaturated fats, all which are great warriors against free radicals, which have been shown to cause cancers and heart disease.